Distribution, publication, and copying in any form are prohibited and subject to damages.

TEN HYPNOSES

Copying, publishing, and sharing with third parties are only permitted with the written consent of the author. Please observe the notes on copyright and usage.

Distribution, publication, and copying in any form are prohibited and subject to damages.

Copying, publishing, and sharing with third parties are only permitted with the written consent of the author. Please observe the notes on copyright and usage.

Distribution, publication, and copying in any form are prohibited and subject to damages.

Ingo Michael Simon

TEN HYPNOSES

37

NEW START AFTER SEPARATION

Copying, publishing, and sharing with third parties are only permitted with the written consent of the author. Please observe the notes on copyright and usage.

Distribution, publication, and copying in any form are prohibited and subject to damages.

© 2024 Ingo Michael Simon
All rights reserved.
Independently published
www.ingosimon.com

Important Notes for Urgent Attention:

The contents of this book are based on the practical experiences of the author with hypnosis applications and psychotherapy in a trance state. Although the author has strived for the utmost care, errors or misunderstandings in the presentation cannot be completely excluded. Therapeutic work with people and the application of hypnosis are solely the responsibility of the hypnotist. It cannot be ruled out that parts of this book may be misunderstood or that the application of a presented procedure may cause an undesirable reaction in the client. The author also assumes no co-responsibility if work with a client is carried out with reference to the statements in this book.

The Author:

Ingo Michael Simon studied psychology and education and is a hypnotherapist with practices in southwestern Germany and Switzerland. With the help of hypnosis-supported psychotherapy, he primarily treats people with persistent psychological conditions. His practice focuses on anxiety disorders, pathological compulsions, and psychosomatic illnesses. His therapeutic offerings mainly include classical and modern hypnosis applications and the dreamland therapy he developed himself.

Copying, publishing, and sharing with third parties are only permitted with the written consent of the author. Please observe the notes on copyright and usage.

Distribution, publication, and copying in any form are prohibited and subject to damages.

INTRODUCTION	6
COPYRIGHT AND USAGE	8
HYPNOSIS 1	10
HYPNOSIS 2	16
HYPNOSIS 3	23
HYPNOSIS 4	29
HYPNOSIS 5	36
HYPNOSIS 6	41
HYPNOSIS 7	47
HYPNOSIS 8	54
HYPNOSIS 9	59
HYPNOSIS 10	65
ALL TITLES IN THE SERIES	72

Copying, publishing, and sharing with third parties are only permitted with the written consent of the author. Please observe the notes on copyright and usage.

Distribution, publication, and copying in any form are prohibited and subject to damages.

Introduction

The series "Ten Hypnoses" is very well known in Germany, Austria, and Switzerland as a collection of texts for therapeutic work and is used by numerous psychotherapeutic practices, doctors, therapists, coaches, and other helping professionals. I am pleased to now be able to offer these texts in other countries as well.

Most therapists have their own methods for inducing and deepening trance as well as for exiting trance. Therefore, I have focused on the main part of the hypnosis. The texts in this book can be integrated as the main part into any hypnosis process. The texts in this collection use various hypnosis techniques. I will not explain these in detail, as I assume that users have the appropriate training. It is also not necessary to understand the exact structure or functioning of the different parts. The texts can simply be read aloud, and they will have their effect.

Decide for yourself which text best suits your client or patient at any given time. You can also combine passages from different texts. It is not about using all ten hypnoses in sequence. It is a selection of possibilities.

Copying, publishing, and sharing with third parties are only permitted with the written consent of the author. Please observe the notes on copyright and usage.

I want to emphasize that books cannot replace therapy. Psychotherapy or other therapeutic treatments involve much more. A careful diagnosis is the necessary basis for deciding on the use of methods, including whether hypnosis or one of my texts should be used. Even in this case, preparatory discussions, follow-up discussions during the session, and of course, a therapeutic concept for the sequence of sessions and the content approaches are essential parts of therapy. This cannot and should not be achieved with a collection of texts.

In any case, I wish you much success in your work and I am pleased if my text templates can contribute in a small way.

Ingo Michael Simon

Distribution, publication, and copying in any form are prohibited and subject to damages.

Copyright and Usage

Copying, publishing, and sharing with third parties is prohibited and only permitted with the written consent of the author. Please observe the following copyright and usage guidelines.

This work has been carefully crafted and created to the best of the author's knowledge and personal experience. It comprises text templates and application guidelines for professional hypnosis sessions. The author is a licensed psychotherapist with extensive experience in psychotherapy, coaching, and personal training using hypnotic techniques and methods. Nevertheless, the author and the publisher assume no liability for the accuracy of information, instructions, and advice, nor for any typographical errors. The author and publisher accept no responsibility or liability for the application of these texts and recommendations with clients or patients, nor for any potential consequences or unexpected reactions. It is expressly noted that the application of therapeutic and advisory techniques and formulations lies solely and entirely within the responsibility of the practitioner. This also applies to adherence to the

Copying, publishing, and sharing with third parties are only permitted with the written consent of the author. Please observe the notes on copyright and usage.

boundaries of legally regulated medical and therapeutic practices. The fact that a book containing action proposals is freely available for sale does not imply that its application with clients or patients is permitted for everyone.

Hypnosis 1

... ... You're here today to say goodbye ... ... You've been separated from someone you lived with, someone you might have wanted to live with for a long time, maybe even for life ... ... Sometimes we have time to prepare for a separation, and sometimes it catches us by surprise ... ... maybe we couldn't or didn't want to see it coming ... ... But in the end, it's always a painful process, even when we're the ones who made the decision to part ways ... ... because something important to us is ending ... ... You know this feeling, you're experiencing it right now ... ... But today, you can do something that will help you let go while still holding on to loving memories ... ... Memories that can help you look back on the past with affection and, at the same time, carry those experiences and memories with you as you move forward on new paths ... ... Remembering, letting go, and moving forward ... ... So today, you'll think back to honor what you shared ... ... to release anything unresolved if there is anything unresolved ... ... and to say what was left unsaid ... ... or simply what you still want to say ... ...

… … When you're in a trance, images and thoughts become friendly suggestions and support for your subconscious and your body, which will respond in harmony with the images you envision … … Perhaps you already knew this because you've learned about hypnosis or researched how and why it works … … or maybe you're surprised and intrigued to hear and experience that this is indeed how it works … … If you think about it, you'll understand that positive and constructive changes in your well-being are most possible when you can let go of disruptive thoughts and feelings and replace them with new, constructive ones … … And this is absolutely possible … … Maybe you're already curious to see how this works … … It's even possible to activate a strength within you that will help you regain a state of inner and outer freedom permanently … … So, let's begin … … You'll think back today to honor what you shared … … to let go of anything unresolved if there's anything unresolved … … and to say what was left unsaid … … or simply what you still want to say … …

… … Deep within you, you have photos of everyone you know … … like a huge album in your memory … … a gallery of your life so far … … All situations and events … … all experiences ... ... even wishes and fantasies are deeply stored within you ... ... and whenever you think of a specific event or person, you can hold a fitting photo of it in your hand ... ... Now, find a photo of the person from whom you are now separated ... [If possible, address more specifically: a photo of your husband ... a photo of your wife ...] ... ... This photo shows you a typical image, as you most often experienced this person ... ... You look at the photo ... ... and memories awaken within you ... ... You recall what it was like when you first met ... ... perhaps just a brief moment of attention that brought you together ... ... or maybe it was fate that brought you together ... ... The images of memory awaken ... ... It's as if you're visiting that past time ... ... reliving how it was back then ... ...

... ... Then, find a photo from stormy and challenging times ... ... This photo shows you that you've experienced a lot together ... ... there were arguments and disagreements ... ... perhaps openly expressed ... ... or silently within you ... ... But then you managed, and better times came again ... ... but eventually, you drifted apart ... ...

... ... Now, find a photo from the best time you spent together ... ... This photo comes to life on its own ... ... as if you could dive back into that time … … You're a visitor to that time and let the mood of those days wash over you once more … … You immerse yourself and feel again the beautiful feelings of shared experiences, of good times … … Perhaps every time was beautiful in its own way … … Everything has its purpose, and every challenge teaches us something … … Look at everything calmly and enjoy those good times … … those wonderful experiences … … If you wish, choose a special moment … … and take your time to look at it again … … Let all the feelings and moods simply be … … All of this is a part of you … … [Now give about a minute of silence, then continue.] … …

+++ Option 1: The client initiated the breakup +++

… … Then you come across a special photo … … one that best shows you why you decided to end the relationship … … It appears on its own … … Accept it, no matter what this photo shows … … Perhaps you recognize a reason you already knew … … or discover another important reason … … something that led you to decide you could no longer continue this relationship … … You associate this with a deep inner feeling … … Let this feeling be fully present … … Now, as you focus on your feeling, you can sense that you made a decision against the relationship and for yourself ... ... There's certainly something you'd like to say ... ... You can do this now, deep inside, just for yourself ... ... quietly and silently ... ... Take your time to say everything you need to until you hear my voice again ... ... [Now, wait for about 2-3 minutes in silence.] ... ...

+++ **End of Option 1** +++

+++ **Option 2: The partner of the client initiated the breakup** +++

... ... Then you come across a special photo ... ... one that best shows you why this breakup had to happen ... ... It appears on its own ... ... Accept it, no matter what this photo shows ... ... Perhaps you recognize a connection or a main cause you already knew ... ... or discover another connection ... ... something that led to or contributed to the end of the relationship ... ... You couldn't stop it, and it wasn't your fault ... ... You associate this with a deep inner feeling ... ... Let this feeling be fully present ... ... Now, as you focus on your feeling, you can sense that the breakup was painful ... ... yet new possibilities arise from it for you ... ... There's certainly something you'd like to say ... ... You can do this now, deep inside, just for yourself ... ... quietly and silently ... ... Take your time to say everything you need to until you hear my voice again ... ... [Now, wait for about 2-3 minutes in silence.] ... ...

+++ **End of Option 2** +++

... ... You can now hear my voice again because I'm still here with you ... ... You've used this time to say or express deep within yourself whatever you needed to say ... ... If you need another moment, take it ... ... continue speaking inwardly ... ... In a few moments, we'll move on ... ... [Give the client another half-minute, then continue reading.] ... ...

... ... Now that you've had the chance to say what was important ... ... it's time to say goodbye ... ... to say farewell and slowly prepare to return to your waking life ... ... Now it's time to move on ... ... You're moving forward on your own path now because that's what truly matters ... ...

Hypnosis 2

… … You've decided to leave this ended relationship behind, to let go today, and to be free again … … You want to rediscover a feeling you once had, in a time long before this relationship, when you were single … … There was a time when you didn't even know you would one day be in a relationship with this person … … back then, you didn't even know them … … The good thing is that this earlier time can help you today … … because if you can recall a time when you were without a relationship and felt good, that feeling still exists within you … … and you know exactly … … There truly was such a time … … whether it was long or short doesn't matter … … You could be happy without a relationship, especially without this relationship that has just ended … … So you can do it again … …

… … Now, go on an inner journey … … a journey through the timeline of your life … … through the images of your memories and the feelings of your life … … Maybe you remember many events in your life well, and it's like a film running backward … … or it's like a journey through a long tunnel, going so quickly it feels like flying or riding a train, and you just let yourself drift … … back to a time when you were single and felt good … … There was this time before the breakup, before the relationship … … It wasn't always there … … There was a time when you didn't even think about the possibility of this relationship because it wasn't even in sight, and you didn't feel like anything was missing … … and on your journey, you're getting closer and closer to this time … … It's as if you're skipping over the time of this relationship … … It's as if you're jumping back to a completely different time … … You don't have to try hard; you don't have to do anything special or come up with any specific memories … … Just imagine that you're arriving at the time before this relationship … … a time when you had no relationship at all and felt good … … Maybe you don't have to travel back very far … … or maybe you have to go back many years … … maybe even to your youth … … That's possible too, and it's easy because it doesn't matter when or how long that free time lasted … … It's just about getting there … … now … … in images … … or simply in your imagination, in your feelings … … and now you're there … …

… … Now, linger in that earlier time … … feel the vibe of that time … … the freedom and openness to life … … That was normal for you back then … … freedom and openness … … That was entirely normal and natural … … Take a look around in your memory … … See where you are … … in what time of your life … … Check how old you were when everything was still good … … when you were still free and thus happy … … See where you are, where your journey has taken you … … and then fully immerse yourself in these images … … or fully in the thought that you've really arrived in this free past … … and dive into the certainty that you're really there, in that good time … … You're back in your thoughts in that free time … … You're back with inner images, with images before your inner eye in that free time … … You're back with your feeling in that free time … … and the good and strong feelings from back then come alive … … It's your old self-confidence coming back … … You feel your self-confidence within you … … It wakes up and becomes strong again … … a lively and strong self-confidence … … Your old spirit of freedom is reactivated … … You feel this old desire for freedom growing stronger … … Your desire for freedom … … the spirit and freedom within you … … a good feeling of freedom for you ... ... and there are more strengths ... ... another strong and helpful feeling now awakens within you ... ... a feeling that was strong back then and now wakes up again ... ... a feeling or ability that helps you overcome the breakup ... ... an ability that makes you strong and free at the same time ... ... Your strengths are now activated and they embed deeply within you, so you can use them anytime, always ... ...

... ... It's as if you can suddenly grasp and hold on to self-confidence, the desire for freedom, and many strengths again ... ... And you really can ... ... You feel these helpful feelings in your body, so you can carry them with you ... ... and filled with your strengths, which are stronger than any guilt or sadness, you go on another journey ... ... You embark on a journey into the future with a complete sense of freedom ... ...

+++ Option 1: The client initiated the breakup +++

... ... It's as if you're traveling through a time tunnel from the past towards the future ... ... filled with your strengths and completely free, you travel to the present and beyond the present into the future ... ... into a truly wonderful future

… … maybe a few days or weeks ahead … … and there you stop, in a free and near future … … You've let go of all self-blame in this time; you've overcome feelings of guilt … … You've realized and understood that you had to make this decision because it was right for you and your sense of well-being … … In this free future, you have a content and self-determined life … …

You shape your life with freedom and joy … … You see what it's like to live easily and naturally without this relationship … … without this partner, whom you now truly let go of … … In this future, you feel your self-confidence and your freedom … … You feel your potential, which guides you safely and easily through your life … … You're completely free and happy … … You're completely free and happy … …

+++ **End of Option 1** +++

+++ **Option 2: The partner of the client initiated the breakup** +++

… … It's as if you're traveling through a time tunnel from the past towards the future … … filled with your strengths and completely free, you travel to the present and beyond the present into the future ... ... into a truly wonderful future ... ... maybe a few days or weeks ahead ... ... and there you stop, in a free and near future ... ... You've long since overcome the shock of the breakup ... ... You've long since let go ... ... You've realized and understood that you cannot hold on to what is ending, and you've recognized and understood that it's better this way ... ... that the breakup was a step towards your freedom and self-determination ... ... In this free future, you have a content and self-determined life ... ...

You shape your life with freedom and joy ... ... You see what it's like to live easily and naturally without this relationship ... ... without this partner, whom you now truly let go of ... ... In this future, you feel your self-confidence and your freedom ... ... You feel your potential, which guides you safely and easily through your life ... ... You're completely free and happy ... ... You're completely free and happy ... ...

+++ **End of Option 2** +++

... ... Filled with this strength, with the good feeling of freedom and the freedom to shape your life, you can now return calmly to the present ... ... to finally leave the past behind in the present, in your waking life, and to walk your path ... ... free and self-determined ... ... You can do this, and you will do this because you are independent and strong ... ... You look forward and anticipate your new life in freedom ... ... You're free ... ... You're truly free ... ...

Hypnosis 3

… … Today, you're experiencing a special trance for inner liberation and a true new beginning … … and you'll reach this trance very quickly … …

… … Today, you're experiencing a special trance for inner liberation and a true new beginning … … and this trance brings a new and good feeling of life … …

… … Today, you're experiencing a special trance for inner liberation and a true new beginning … … and the following suggestions will help you with this … …

… … Today, you're experiencing a special trance for inner liberation and a true new beginning … … and that's why you're also ready to accept all suggestions … …

… … All thoughts and memories of the shared time, you now let go of them, just let them go … … and you become free and open to a new path … …

… … All thoughts and memories of the shared time, you now let go of them, just let them go … … and with letting go, you feel inner freedom … …

… … All thoughts and memories of the shared time, you now let go of them, just let them go … … and you only look forward … …

… … All thoughts and memories of the shared time, you now let go of them, just let them go … … and all inner tensions dissolve and freedom begins … …

… … You're free inside, and you're starting anew … … Now … …

+++ Option 1: The client initiated the breakup +++

… … The calmness of your body becomes a feeling of security on your new path … … and that's why it's so easy for you to let go of this relationship now … …

… … The calmness of your body becomes a feeling of security on your new path … … and that's why you let go of all feelings of guilt today … …

… … The calmness of your body becomes a feeling of security on your new path … … and with that, a new constructive time begins for you … … now … …

… … The calmness of your body becomes a feeling of security on your new path … … and that's why you're now starting your new life … … now … …

… … You're free inside, and you're starting anew … … Now … …

+++ End of Option 1 +++

+++ Option 2: The partner of the client initiated the breakup +++

… … The calmness within you becomes a feeling of security and freedom on your new path … … and that's why it's so easy for you to let go of this relationship now … …

… … The calmness within you becomes a feeling of security and freedom on your new path … … and that's why you let go of all accusations and any anger today … …

… … The calmness within you becomes a feeling of security and freedom on your new path … … and with that, a new constructive time begins for you … … now … …

… … The calmness within you becomes a feeling of security and freedom on your new path … … and that's why you're now starting your new life … … now … …

… … You're free inside, and you're starting anew … … Now … …

+++ **End of Option 2** +++

… … You're filled with a deep feeling of inner freedom and healing peace … … and this peace spreads throughout your body … …

… … You're filled with a deep feeling of inner freedom and healing peace … … and this peace is a balm for body, mind, and soul … …

… … You're filled with a deep feeling of inner freedom and healing peace … … and this state heals all hurts and emotional wounds … …

… … You're filled with a deep feeling of inner freedom and healing peace … … and in this peace, you can let go of everything and be free … …

… … You're free inside, and you're starting anew … … Now … …

...... Now you can truly walk your own path, step by step ...... because in this deep relaxation, you've truly freed yourself ......

...... Now you can truly walk your own path, step by step ...... because you've really left the old behind ......

...... Now you can truly walk your own path, step by step ...... because you're really ready for a new path ......

...... Now you can truly walk your own path, step by step ...... because you're free, independent, and strong ......

...... You're free inside, and you're starting anew ...... Now ......

...... Now feel the deep calm of the trance and also feel the deep sense of liberation and freedom within you ...... and this feeling is your starting point into independence ......

...... Now feel the deep calm of the trance and also feel the deep sense of liberation and freedom within you ...... and this feeling carries you safely and securely ......

...... Now feel the deep calm of the trance and also feel the deep sense of liberation and freedom within you ...... and this feeling makes you confident and strong ......

... ... Feel and enjoy the deep calm of the trance ... ... Feel and enjoy the freedom ... ... Feel and enjoy your new path in life ... ...

Hypnosis 4

Guidance for the Session

In this hypnosis session, a self-hypnosis trigger will be trained. A self-hypnosis trigger is a signal that initiates the trance state. It allows even a beginner to continue practicing self-hypnosis at home. Of course, they can use simple suggestions that are easy to remember and that we should prepare, or they can work with simple visualizations. Triggered self-hypnosis is an excellent tool to give the client a task and to support the therapy. This way, the time between sessions in the office is not without therapy, but it is continued at home. Completely self-directed self-hypnosis without a trigger is also learnable, but it requires much time and practice. Setting up the trigger is a relatively simple task and naturally eases the burden on the client, as I do not want to impose the training of self-directed self-hypnosis on them. Despite some concerns, I assert that there is no problem in teaching a client simple triggered self-hypnosis. It is no more dangerous than meditation, autogenic training, or yoga. People survive these activities at home unscathed as well. I've had numerous patients in my practice who not only handled self-hypnosis well but also enjoyed it. And if a patient enjoys doing self-hypnosis, no matter how simple the suggestions may seem, that's a great way to support compliance. Discuss the process once before hypnosis and give the client a brief, bullet-point list of the steps for self-hypnosis so they have a small guide.

+++ **End of Guidance** +++

… … You've been feeling lonely since your breakup … … And it's challenging to break free from this feeling and look ahead … … Self-hypnosis can help you overcome the toughest moments and quickly reach a sense of connection to yourself … … In self-hypnosis, you can feel much more clearly than in a waking state that you are deeply connected with yourself, so deeply that you cannot feel any loneliness within … … This way, you can also let go of the feeling of loneliness even when no one else is around … … It's actually quite simple, and I'll show you how … … You'll learn how to do it now … … Now that you're in a trance, you can also easily learn how to do self-hypnosis … …

… … I'll show you how to enter the trance … … There's a trigger, a code word, that brings you into a trance … … It's called … … Ridola … [Emphasize the first syllable: Ri-dola.] … … At home, make yourself comfortable and close your eyes, just like here … … and then whisper this trance word over and over until you become sleepy, and that happens quickly … … You'll become sleepy very quickly when you whisper … … Ridola – Ridola – Ridola - Ridola – Ridola – Ridola … … and with that, you'll already reach a pleasant trance, just like here … … Your trigger … … Ridola … … will imprint deeply into your subconscious now … … so you can easily use it whenever you want to enter a trance … …

… … Then, you go deeper into the trance because in the deeper trance, there's no sense of loneliness; instead, you're very close to yourself … … In deep trance, you're very close to yourself, and this closeness leaves no room for loneliness … … You reach this deeper trance by whispering ten times … … I'm sinking deeper and deeper, towards the silence … … You just whisper … … I'm sinking once, deeper and deeper, towards the silence … … I'm sinking twice, deeper and deeper, towards the silence … … I'm sinking three times, deeper and deeper, towards the silence, and so on … … until you finally reach ten and whisper … … I'm sinking ten times, deeper and deeper, towards the silence … … and with that, you enter this deeper trance where you never feel lonely but always connected … … connected with yourself … … The trance you reach is truly deep and pleasant … … just like here … … You're in complete safety … … and you can control everything yourself … … It's very simple because you're learning it now … …

[For deepening and the main part, I recommend counting with the suggestions … once … twice, etc. The advantage is that the client is not distracted by wondering how many times they've repeated the suggestion. It's not really about repeating ten times; in trance, the client can more easily stay on track this way. You can also say all ten repetitions out loud. After all, this hypnosis is also suggestive. It's not just a self-hypnosis training session, but a hypnosis session.]

… … Then comes the main part of your self-hypnosis … … The main part helps you, above all, to turn the feeling of loneliness, when it's particularly strong, into a sense of connection … … Connection with yourself, because you're always there … … In this part, you work with a suggestion that frees you ... ... You simply repeat it ten times ... ... Ten times you whisper ... ...

+++ **Option 1: The client initiated the breakup** +++

... ... I walk my path and embrace myself with love ... ... While counting ... ... You say ... ... I walk my path once and embrace myself with love ... ... I walk my path twice and embrace myself with love ... ... I walk my path three times and embrace myself with love ... ... until you reach ten and finally say and feel ... ... I walk my path ten times and embrace myself with love ... ... and then you feel that you're never lonely within yourself ... ... You feel connected with yourself and your memories ... ...

+++ **End of Option 1** +++

+++ **Option 2: The partner of the client initiated the breakup** +++

... ... I find connection and stability deep within me ... ... While counting ... ... You say ... ... I find connection and stability deep within me once ... ... I find connection and stability deep within me twice ... ... I find connection and stability deep within me three times ... ... until you reach ten and say ... ... I find connection and stability deep within me ten times ... ... and then you feel that you're never lonely within yourself ... ... You feel connected with yourself and your beautiful memories ... ... with your deep strength that always carries and guides you ... ... always ... ...

+++ End of Option 2 +++

... ... To wake yourself up again, imagine a cold wind blowing ... ... Then you say ... ... I'm waking up now and feeling good ... ... and then count out loud and clearly to three and open your eyes ... ... It's very easy ... ... So, once again ... ... To wake up, imagine a cold wind blowing and you say ... ... I'm waking up now and feeling good – One – Two – Three ... ... and then open your eyes because you're awake ... ... It's very simple, and you can try it later again ... ...

... ... You've learned how to do self-hypnosis ... ... You know everything you need to know ... ... You can use it from now on whenever you feel particularly lonely, to quickly feel a sense of connection ... ... and loneliness fades away because it's no longer possible ... ... You've learned to enter a trance quickly with your trance word, and you know how to proceed ... ... Your trance word ... Ridola ... brings you into trance, which you deepen with the words … … I'm sinking deeper and deeper, towards the silence … … Then comes your suggestion … … {Insert the chosen suggestion from the main part here} … … This suggestion banishes loneliness … … At the end of the self-hypnosis session, imagine a cold wind and say … I'm waking up now and feeling good – One – Two – Three … …

Hypnosis 5

... ... You want to start a new chapter in your life today ... ... and to do that, you want to let go of the past and leave it behind ... ... The relationship that has just ended, you want to and will give it to the past today and completely free yourself from it ... ... It's about keeping the good and happy memories and storing the entire time as an experience ... ... That's possible ... ... because every experience can help you grow and mature ... ... Every life experience allows you to make good and appropriate decisions today and in the future ... ... Today, you align your inner energy and thoughts in such a way that you can start anew today ... ... into a free and self-determined life ... ... with the help of a very special thought ... ...

... ... Perhaps you already know that a single thought can change your whole mood ... ... This is really possible ... ... When we think of something that touches us emotionally, our inner tension and heartbeat change immediately ... ... because the body and feelings react to it ... ... A constructive thought can therefore send our organism on a constructive path and accompany and guide it there ... ... and that's what it's all about ... ... a constructive path ... ... A good thought ... ... a special sentence, can change everything for the better ... ... You can use such a special thought as an affirmation ... ... An affirmation is like a guiding thought that always helps you ... ... You can use such a phrase over and over to find the best path for your free and self-determined life ... ... and it's much easier than you think ... ...

... ... Enjoy the trance ... ... It has a calming effect on your thoughts and your body, helping you relax both your thoughts and your body ... ... and physical relaxation is something you can really use ... ... because it leads to your thoughts and feelings becoming calmer, and you're already becoming freer inside ... ... But there's much more ... ... The calmness of the trance is like a starting point for a new life ... ... for a completely new chapter that leads you onto a free path ... ... In this calmness, you can already experience the inner separation from the past ... ... today ... ... now ... ... To do this, focus on a constructive thought of letting go and freedom ... ... You can firmly anchor this thought today and then use it again and again for yourself ... ... like a belief ... ... like a creed ... ... in trance and also in a fully awake state, this thought will help you … … and who knows, maybe it sounds exactly like your inner voice … … The affirmation you're about to hear will become the one thought that guides you now and always on the path to freedom … … You hear your inner voice saying … … {5-10 seconds pause} … …

+++ **Option 1: The client initiated the breakup** +++

… … I made the decision to break up for my freedom and constructive path, and I continue on this path with a good feeling … …

+++ **End of Option 1** +++

+++ **Option 2: The partner of the client initiated the breakup** +++

… … I embrace my new freedom and find new and constructive impulses for my personal journey every day … …

+++ **End of Option 2** +++

… … And now simply enjoy the calmness because this will quickly make the affirmation you've heard become your inner attitude … … so the affirmation you've heard becomes the attitude of your inner self … … because you make this thought the most important of all thoughts … … because you've heard it in trance and thus made it your special creed … … a creed that expresses your intention, your goal, and your will … … but even more than that … … It expresses your possibilities … … This affirmation expresses what is truly possible and what you're really ready for … …

… … Your freedom affirmation now acts as a deep-seated attitude of your inner self and your decisions … … as a deep inner attitude that you feel clearly … … The freedom affirmation becomes your own voice inside … …

+++ Option 1: The client initiated the breakup +++

… … I made the decision to break up for my freedom and constructive path, and I continue on this path with a good feeling … …

+++ End of Option 1 +++

+++ Option 2: The partner of the client initiated the breakup +++

... ... I embrace my new freedom and find new and constructive impulses for my personal journey every day ... ...

+++ End of Option 2 +++

... ... And now let the impact of your new and stable inner attitude fully unfold ... ... It's really easy because you can trust that your new belief will stabilize in this trance and already make you feel free deep inside ... ... free for your new and self-determined life ... ... free for new paths ... ... free for new decisions ... ... free for your path ... ...

Hypnosis 6

… … Surely you know that people say they listen to their inner voice … … Perhaps you've said this yourself many times and actually done it … … Usually, the inner voice refers to a feeling … … the gut feeling … … When we listen to our gut feeling, we say it's the inner voice … … And that's true because our deep feelings are always felt in our bodies … … We feel them most clearly in our gut … … This gut feeling always shows us the right path … … It shows us what's good and right for us … … and it can also warn us … … of mistakes and dangers … … Exactly these deep-seated feelings … … these hidden emotions come to the surface and show themselves as a bodily sensation … … more precisely, as a gut feeling … … or as tension … … or a tingling sensation … … Surely you know your personal gut feeling … … or at least how your deep feelings show themselves … … But you can also perceive the inner voice in another way … … You can actually hear it, just like you hear me now … … maybe even just as loudly and clearly … … What you need for this is calmness and openness … … Now, follow my voice and in a few moments, find the voice within you and listen to what it has to say ... ... Follow me closely ... ...

... ... Now, focus only on the music you hear ... ... Listen to the music and let it become clear ... ... Hear only the music; everything else is secondary now ... ... Only the music matters now ... ... Now, focus entirely on the music here in the room ... ... until you hear my voice again ... ... [Now, wait for about a minute in silence] ... ...

... ... Now, focus absolutely and exclusively on my voice ... ... Focus absolutely and exclusively on my voice ... ... Let it become increasingly clear ... ... Only my voice counts now ... ... Only my voice matters now ... ... only my voice ... ... good ... ... That's right ... ... [Now, wait for about a minute in silence] ... ...

... ... Now, take in the sounds of the room we're in ... ... Notice as many sounds as possible ... ... Let the music fade into the background now ... ... Let it become quiet and only notice the sounds in this room ... ... until you hear my voice again ... ... [Now, wait for about a minute in silence] ... ...

... ... Now, take your hearing further out and listen to the sounds of the house ... ... Now, only listen to the sounds of the house ... ... the sounds outside of our room ... ... now only the sounds outside of our room matter ... ... until you hear my voice again ... ... [Now, wait for about a minute in silence] ... ...

... ... Now, go even further outside and listen to the sounds outside the house and around the house ... ... Now, only the sounds from outside matter and let them become very clear ... ... Only the outside sounds are important now ... ... Listen to the sounds outside ... ... until you hear my voice again ... ... [Now, wait for about a minute in silence] ... ...

... ... Now, go way up and even listen above the clouds ... ... It's possible ... ... Hear the sounds of the sky ... ... Listen to the wind high above ... ... Hear the drifting clouds high above ... ... Listen to what's beyond the clouds ... ... Hear beyond the clouds ... ... until you hear my voice again ... ... [Now, wait for about a minute in silence] ... ...

... ... And now, listen deep into the universe ... ... Wander with your hearing into infinity ... ... Now, hear the sounds of infinity ... ... Let your hearing go far into space ... ... further and further away ... ... Hear the sounds of infinity ... ... until you hear my voice again … … [Now, wait for about a minute in silence] … …

… … Now, feel the vastness of the universe … … Feel the openness and infinity of space and enjoy the sounds of infinity … … Maybe you hear a symphony … … Maybe it's the wonderful silence of infinity … … or it's completely different, wonderful sounds and perceptions … … so far out … … way out there … … infinitely far away … … [Another 30 seconds of silence] … …

… … Enjoy the openness and vastness of infinity … … Just be there and allow every perception … … Everything you can hear belongs to you … … Everything you can feel belongs to you … … Everything, absolutely everything belongs to you … … only to you … …

+++ Option 1: The client initiated the breakup +++

… You ended your relationship … … It was your decision, and it was a good and right decision for you … … Now you're wondering how things will go on and how they will unfold … … Just ask this question into infinity … … The universe hears your question … … What's next? … …

+++ End of Option 1 +++

+++ Option 2: The partner of the client initiated the breakup +++

… … Your partner ended the relationship … … It wasn't your decision; you had to accept it as it was … … Now you're wondering how things will go on and how they will unfold … … Trust in the vastness and wisdom of the universe and look into infinity now … … Just ask this question into infinity … … The universe hears your question … … What's next? … …

+++ End of Option 2 +++

… [Please read the following section of focusing quickly. Make sure to read really quickly and without pauses and emphasize the bold words clearly!] …

… … Now come immediately and quickly back to this room, right now, and now listen deeply into your body. Bring all your attention deep into your body now and listen to your inner voice. Listen to your inner voice now … … [Now, wait for about a minute in silence] … …

… … Good … … Whatever your inner voice says to you, just let it be … … Let the words you've heard from your inner voice simply be there … … Maybe you understood them and know why your inner voice is telling you this … …

But if you can't make sense of what you heard, just accept it anyway … … It will have its effect, and the words you've heard will help you be closer to yourself … … You're already much closer to yourself than before … … closer than you think … … Focus on your body and feel the closeness to yourself … … That's good … … That's right … …

Hypnosis 7

Guidance for the Session

An anchor (or trigger) is a stimulus that produces a specific feeling or triggers a specific thought. It is a signal perceived by the client that then initiates an inner process. The set anchor then replaces the suggestion. In everyday life, a client can trigger a desired state with an anchor or trigger, even without a trance state. Various stimuli can be used as anchors/triggers. I work with the following options, which I also use in the series "Ten Hypnoses":

- Body anchors (closing the hand, pressing the thumb pad ...)
- Visual anchors (symbols, word cards ...)
- Auditory anchors (signal sounds like phone rings, melodies ...)
- Olfactory anchors (essential oils ...)
- Tactile anchors (hand comforter, talisman ...)

I also distinguish between peri-hypnotic and post-hypnotic anchors. Peri-hypnotic anchors are those mainly used during hypnosis, where the therapist sets up the anchor and then repeatedly triggers it as an addition to the suggestions and visualizations. Post-hypnotic anchors are primarily set up for the time after the session, so the client can help themselves with it.

+++ **End of Guidance** +++

… … Today, we'll place an anchor … … An anchor is a simple tool that helps you let go of the past and focus on the present … … just like an anchor that holds a ship in place even in storms and high waves, your anchor will help you stay in the present and be free … … especially when you think the past is catching up with you … … And you should always be able to carry your anchor with you … … it will first help you let go of the past … … and then it will constantly ensure that you experience the present as an opportunity for a fresh start and constructive development … … You have this important goal-oriented thought that tells you … … I am free and open to a new and self-determined life … … You want to firmly anchor this thought to truly feel free and move forward ... ...

[Have a card ready with the inscription "I am free and open to a new and self-determined life" and discuss before hypnosis that you will give the client the card during the session. They don't need to open their eyes. Announce a touch briefly before handing over the card, and then touch the client's hand with it so they can grasp it. Just follow the instructions in the text!] ...

... ... Now you just need to relax and feel good, focus on the future ... ... now, at this very moment ... ... It's probably very easy for you now; you likely feel relaxed and free, after all, you're in a trance and quite relaxed ... ... and in relaxation, you automatically feel freer ... ... Now you feel relaxation and inner freedom ... ... Now you can constructively look ahead ... ... Now you can focus on your future and imagine having a good and self-determined life ... ... Pay attention to your feelings, focus on yourself ... ... Feel yourself ... ... The more you manage to focus on yourself now, in this moment, just on the feeling of relaxation ... ... in this very moment ... ... the better you can now also feel that you are inwardly free and truly open and ready for your new self-determined life ... ... Now you don't have to worry about anything ... ... Now you don't have to achieve anything ... ... Now you have peace ... ...

... ... Now, in deep relaxation, you can encounter yourself openly, let go of the past and the past relationship, and feel free ... ... It's much easier now than ever ... ... You accept yourself in this moment and are free ... ... The more clearly you can feel relaxation now, the better you can feel free within yourself ... ... So feel the relaxation and accept yourself ... ... Now ... ... Now it's happening ... ... You can feel calm and freedom ... ... Now I'm giving you the card in your hand ... ... [Touch the client's hand and hand them the card. They can keep their eyes closed.] ... ... Feel the card in your hand ... ... You know what it says ... ... It says: I am free and open to a new and self-determined life ... ... You think about this sentence, about this attitude ... ... You feel that you are feeling good now ... ... You're completely free now and feel good ... ... and now you focus on yourself ... ... you intend, as it says on the card, to feel free ... ... to actively and joyfully shape your life ... ... The card reminds you that you can feel good, just like you feel good now, because it's always and everywhere possible ... ... especially when memories or longing arise ... ... The card helps you because whenever you carry it with you, you feel as safe as you do now ... ...

+++ Option 1: The client initiated the breakup +++

... ... when you carry it with you, you feel as good as you do now because you remember how good you feel now ... ... your whole body remembers, your entire organism remembers the relaxation and stays this relaxed ... ... your anchor helps you with this ... ... just like today ... ... the card helps you with this ... ... You feel good and know that the breakup was the right decision for you ... ... You know that you chose yourself, your freedom, your path ... ... and that's good because you are the most important person in your life ... ... This card in your hands is your anchor ... ... the anchor that holds you in calmness ... ... the anchor that prevents you from drifting into despair ... ... You don't fall into melancholy; you stay in the constructive present ... ... you stay in this constructive feeling that you feel now because your anchor holds you there ... ... Your anchor keeps you in the present ... ...

+++ End of Option 1 +++

+++ Option 2: The partner of the client initiated the breakup +++

… … when you carry it with you, you feel safe within yourself … … your whole body remembers, your entire organism remembers the deep sense of safety, and you feel exactly that feeling … … your anchor helps you with this … … just like today … … the card helps you with this … … You feel good and let go of the relationship … … now and every day, and you start anew … … You let go of anger and resentment … … You overcome disappointments and hurts … … This card in your hands is your anchor … … the anchor that frees you over and over again … … the anchor that prevents you from drifting into despair or anger … … You stay in the constructive present … … you stay in this constructive feeling that you feel now because your anchor leads you there again and again … … Your anchor makes you free … …

+++ End of Option 2 +++

… … You can carry the card with you every day … … and whenever you feel like the past or melancholy and sadness are catching up or could trap you, you can hold it in your hand and read what it says … … I am free and open to a new and self-determined life … … and immediately you feel more calmness and the sense of freedom deep within … … just like now … … exactly like now … … even if you just hold the card in your hand or touch it without reading it, you'll clearly feel the liberation and positive energy … … just like today, every day exactly like today … …

Hypnosis 8

... ... You're here for a reason today ... ... You've often and repeatedly dealt with the end of your relationship lately ... ... you've tried to let go internally and leave this time behind to start anew ... ... you've tried to let go of old feelings of guilt and a bad conscience because these feelings no longer help you ... ... They've only been blocking you, and even working on them often feels like a brake ... ... Today, it can be different because today you don't have to deal with it at all ... ... Today, you can just let things happen and maybe you'll be surprised at how well that works and how much it can help you ... ... So now allow yourself to do nothing ... ... and become free in the process ... ...

... ... Doing nothing means simply following a mental image ... ... imagining a simple picture that I'll describe to you in a few moments ... ... Then you don't need to do anything else; you don't need to make any effort to become free and overcome the breakup ... ... You simply imagine the picture, and that happens automatically as I speak about it ... ... The better you manage to just look at this picture and nothing else, the faster you'll reach your goal … … or rather … … The goal will reach you … … So just follow my words, which will guide and lead you … … Let my voice show you this pleasant and free path … … and experience the unique relief and freedom that you'll find in a simple but very meaningful picture … …

… … So far, it's been like this … … You've felt guilty, you've had a bad conscience, and you've blamed yourself for the end of the relationship … … But from now on, this is how it's going to be … … This is your path … …

[When stating the goal, feel free to place your palm on the client's solar plexus and then remove it. It's not necessary but helps a lot because it "anchors" the goal statement. Of course, you can also incorporate energetic techniques into the hypnosis. Make sure not to repeat the goal.]

+++ **Option 1: The client initiated the breakup** +++
… … Complete freedom from feelings of guilt, freedom, and openness for new paths in your life … …

+++ **End of Option 1** +++

+++ **Option 2: The partner of the client initiated the breakup** +++

… … Complete freedom from personal guilt and from anger and resentment, freedom, and openness for new paths in your life … …

+++ **End of Option 2** +++

… … Now, direct your attention to your breath and feel how your breath flows in and out … … in and out … … [Please follow the client's breathing rhythm!] … … in and out … … in and out … … and now continue to pay attention to the flow of your breath and imagine a small golden light sphere in your body … … in your solar plexus … … a small sphere of pure golden light … … pleasantly warm and beautiful … … Focus entirely on the image of this light sphere and let it grow slightly larger with each breath … … with each breath, the light sphere grows a little larger … … Let your breath flow calmly … … breathe calmly in and out … … and with each breath, the golden light sphere in your inner center becomes a little bigger … … and bigger … … [in the client's breathing rhythm] … … and bigger … … good … … The light sphere is now as big as a ball and continues to expand … … Its edge gently moves outside your body … … and the sphere of golden light grows bigger and bigger … … and now surrounds your body from the outside more and more … … in a few breaths, your whole body will be surrounded by this light sphere … … just a few more breaths, then it will be complete … … Your body is now fully surrounded by this light sphere … … You are at the center of the golden sphere, which continues to grow larger and larger … … With each breath, it expands further … … until it surrounds the building you're in and continues to grow … … The larger the light sphere becomes, the faster it grows … … and soon it reaches above the clouds … … and encompasses the entire earth, becoming the atmosphere of golden light … … a huge sphere of golden light surrounds the entire earth … … and at the center of this light sphere, you stand, breathing deeply … … You are the center of the light sphere … … You are, at this moment, the center of the world … … the center of the world … …

… … Continue to breathe calmly and steadily … … calmly and steadily … … and imagine the light sphere growing smaller with each exhale … … with each breath, it becomes a bit smaller … … always on the exhale … … The sphere gets smaller … … [in the client's breathing rhythm] … … and smaller … … [in the client's breathing rhythm] … … and smaller … … It returns to the clouds and brings the entire power of the universe back to its center ... ... to the center where you stand ... ... The light sphere returns to you ... ... becoming smaller and bringing the power of the earth with it ... ... The sphere still surrounds the building we are in ... ... it passes through the walls and is here in the room, surrounding your entire body, which remains in the center of the golden light sphere ... ... and finally, it is small enough to fit entirely within your body and remain there as a powerful sphere of golden light ... ... in your inner center ... ... in your solar plexus ... ...

... ... Now let your thoughts wander ... ... just let them drift ... ... No thought is important now ... ... There's nothing left to do because everything is already done ... ... Everything is already completed ... ... Let go of the image of the light sphere because the feeling will stay with you ... ... Feel the connection to your body and the surface ... ...

Hypnosis 9

… … Today, I want to accompany you on a very special inner journey … … a journey that takes place in your imagination … … and at the same time in reality, in a very real and true world … … because imagination is more than just creative thinking or dreaming … … Imagination is the liberated potential of our own creativity … … Our imagination can create worlds and let them disappear again, create something new every day, and bring everything to a good end … … But in all dreams and perhaps even unimaginable images, there's always a special truth, a reality that always lies within our imagination and always shapes it … … the truth of our feelings … … because everything we can think of and dream of is an expression of our feelings … … So imagination is emotion turned into an image … … You're going to that place in your imagination where your feelings become helpful images … … images that help you change your life constructively … … You're going to the land of dreams … …

… … In the land of dreams, everything is as you want it to be … … it looks just the way you like it … … Here, you can shape and change everything according to your wishes … … There are no limits here … … So you set out to explore the land of dreams, and you feel that you're exploring your own feelings because everything here is part of your feelings … … Feelings that become images … … and conversely, it works exactly the same … … Every image you imagine becomes a feeling … … You think back to the time of the breakup … … A difficult time … …

+++ Option 1: The client initiated the breakup +++

… … You had felt for a long time that the relationship you were in was no longer right … … Maybe you fought for it for a long time or didn't want to admit that it had to end … … You tried to keep everything together somehow … … maybe because you were still connected to your partner with love … … or because you didn't want to or couldn't accept that the love had already faded … … But then you made the decision to part ways … … It was a tough decision … … and with the memory of it, the sky over the land of dreams turns gray and dark … … Everything here follows your feeling, and the memory of that time makes the sky gray … …

+++ End of Option 1 +++

+++ Option 2: The partner of the client initiated the breakup +++

… … Deep down, you felt that the relationship you were in was no longer right … … Over time, a lot had changed … … Common interests were lost … … Paths diverged … … and maybe you didn't realize for a long time that the two of you, you and your partner, were walking different paths … … Perhaps you only really understood it with the breakup or even later … … Maybe, deep inside, you fought for the relationship for a long time and finally had to realize that it was no longer salvageable … … But you can save yourself, and maybe you'll soon believe that this breakup was the beginning of your rescue … … Maybe it's an unavoidable step, who knows? … … But now it's about taking that step because the breakup has happened … … and you can and will successfully navigate this new chapter of life … … You think back to the time of the breakup … … and with the memory of it, the sky over the land of dreams turns gray and dark … … Everything here follows your feeling, and the memory of that time makes the sky gray … …

+++ **End of Option 2** +++

… … You look up at the gray sky, and then your gaze sweeps across the vast land … … You see meadows and forests, mountains, and valleys, but everything lies in a gray shadow … … Everything looks like a black-and-white film … … It's the feelings of disappointment and inner pain that make everything so gray … … It's the feelings of the painful ending and the fear of what comes next … … But you remember that in the land of dreams, you can create and shape everything the way you can imagine … … and with that, you can also change your feelings … … strictly speaking, it's about regaining pleasant and constructive feelings, because they're always within you … … But the painful and sad feelings cloud the view and your sense of beauty … … just as they cloud the colors here and make everything appear gray … …

… … You close your eyes and take a deep breath to connect with your deepest feelings and with your strength and will to move forward and embrace the new chapter in your life and shape it actively … … Then you open your eyes and look at the ground in front of you … … and there, a small spring appears before your eyes … … Golden water gushes from this spring ... ... and flows over the gray ground, which is touched by the golden color ... ... You watch the spring water flow away ... ... It flows over the ground, deeper into the land of dreams ... ... becomes a stream and then a river that grows wider and wider ... ... and the colors return ... ... The land of dreams is bathed in color again ... ... You see green meadows and forests ... ... Trees and blooming flowers in every imaginable color ... ... Suddenly, the nature of the dreamland is bathed in vibrant colors and shines in radiant splendor ... ... and with these colors, the feeling of life returns to you ... ... You feel hope and confidence again ... ... You feel the drive to act and curiosity ... ... You feel the strength and desire to experience new things and enjoy life ... ...

... ... You keep going, deeper and deeper into the land of dreams to explore ever new landscapes and regions, to experience this beautiful and colorful nature ... ...

... ... On your way to new freedom and a new chapter in the land of dreams, it becomes clear to you that you can walk this same path in your waking life too ... ... because everything you can do here and achieve here, you can also accomplish in your waking life ... ... because everything always begins here … … Everything begins in your feelings … … in the land of dreams … … Is it imagination? … … Maybe … … But the land of dreams is also more than imagination … … It's truth … … It truly exists … … The land of dreams lies deep within you … … It's always been there … … I'm only telling you about it … …

Hypnosis 10

Guidance for the Session

Ideomotorics refers to the phenomenon where our body follows our thoughts and feelings with movements. In everyday life, this following is shown as posture, muscle tension, and movement patterns of a person that naturally change with mood and thoughts. In trance, ideomotoric signals can be used to receive information that the client cannot actively communicate. The subconscious can, for example, answer questions with an agreed-upon finger signal. Of course, ideomotoric reactions can also be used suggestively, for example, with arm levitation and catalepsy. An ideomotoric approach strengthens trust in hypnosis and in one's ability to change and thus promotes therapy.

+++ **End of Guidance** +++

… … You want to start anew internally so that you can also start fresh in the external, in your everyday life … … You've experienced a breakup, and this breakup has cost a lot of energy … … But the time before that was already exhausting, perhaps marked by arguments and conflicts … … Many things were and perhaps remained unspoken … … Then came the day of the breakup, and with it the challenge to begin anew … … because a new chapter in life is beginning … … Your subconscious can help you with this because it's mainly about you aligning yourself with all your strength and energy for this new chapter in your life … … It's like flipping a switch inside … … or like pressing a start button … … I invite your subconscious to work with me and with you … … Your subconscious can and will help you … … here and today … … once and for all … …

… … Imagine for a moment that your subconscious could make your arm feel light … … so light that it rises into the air as if weightless … … If your subconscious can do that, then it can also press your internal reset button and make your fresh start possible and support you … … but your subconscious can do even more … … It can show you that it really does this, that it really presses this reset button … … because only then will your arm become light … … Your arm becomes light and rises up on its own, as soon as your subconscious is ready and willing to support you … … So, imagine your right arm is very light, feather-light, because three thick balloons filled with helium are tied to it ... ... Helium is a very light gas ... ... Three thick helium balloons are tied to your right arm and pull your arm upward ... ... as soon as your subconscious is ready to help you ... ... Your arm becomes lighter and rises ... ... More helium balloons are added, and they are all tied to your wrist ... ... ten balloons are now pulling on your right arm ... ... then twenty balloons, which are pulling and pulling on your right arm ... ... Your arm is being pulled up, higher and higher ... ... Your arm rises into the air ... ... higher and higher, your arm becomes feather-light ... ... Your arm becomes light and rises into the air, rises higher and higher, as if by itself ... ...

[Stay with this. The suggestive connection between the rising arm and the fresh start is already established. The ongoing suggestion of lightness and balloons will eventually cause the arm to move – It will happen!]

... ... There you go ... ... It works ... ... Your arm is floating in the air, and the helium balloons are holding it there ... ... Your arm is held in exactly this position, and it's very easy ... ... Your arm stays up, and that's good ... ... Just open your eyes for a moment, and your arm stays in this position ... ...

Open your eyes and look at your arm; it remains held in exactly this position ... ...

[Always have clients look at the levitating arm for a moment; otherwise, it could be mistaken for a sensory illusion. It's important for the floating arm to be consciously experienced because it strengthens belief in and trust in the possibilities of hypnosis. Don't worry – The arm will stay up. Fracturing is not necessary.]

... ... Now you can close your eyes again ... ... Your arm is held up, it has risen into the air and is held there, and now it becomes stiff like an iron rod ... ... Your arm becomes very firm and stable, very firm and stable ... ... Now your arm becomes firmer and stays up here in the air all by itself ... ... It's easy ... ... Your arm becomes firmer and completely immovable ... ... nothing and no one could move your arm now ... ... I'll show you by pressing against your arm, and it won't give way ... ... Your arm is firm like an iron rod ... ... very firm and stable ... ...

[Press against the arm, which will offer you strong resistance. The client will experience that their arm is indeed cataleptic. But don't overdo it, please! Gentle pressure! The connection between catalepsy and new strength has already been established suggestively. The cataleptic arm "proves" the inner change to the client.]

… … It's done, your arm has risen … … I told your subconscious to only allow this to happen if it was also ready to support your fresh start so that your new beginning will be easy … … and now it's time … … You're ready to start anew; you've overcome the breakup deep inside … … Deep inside, you're already on your new path in life … … very good … …

+++ Option 1: The client initiated the breakup +++

… … You've now achieved a lot … … Now the helium balloons can disappear, and your arm can become heavier again … … Your arm becomes heavy again and slowly sinks back onto the surface … … And as your arm sinks, you let go of the shared time … … You say goodbye internally to your ex-partner and fully embrace your own new path in peace … … As soon as your arm touches the surface, the inner separation is also complete, and you are free because, with that, you let go of the shared time with your ex-partner … … You're ready for your new chapter in life … … Your arm sinks back onto the surface and becomes completely movable again ... ... Your arm is completely movable, and you have full control over your arm ... ... You can move it, including your fingers ... ... [Stay with it until the arm rests relaxed on the surface.] ... ... good ... ... very good ... ...

+++ End of Option 1 +++

+++ Option 2: The partner of the client initiated the breakup +++

... ... You've now achieved a lot ... ... Now the helium balloons can disappear, and your arm can become heavier again ... ... Your arm becomes heavy again and slowly sinks back onto the surface ... ... And as soon as it touches the surface, you feel free because you're letting go of the shared time with your ex-partner ... ... You're ready for your new chapter in life, which you'll navigate confidently and self-determinedly ... ... and as soon as your arm touches the surface, you feel this inner separation and freedom, which feels good ... ... Your arm sinks back onto the surface and becomes completely movable again ... ... Your arm is completely movable, and you have full control over your arm ... ... You can move it, including your fingers ... ... [Stay with it until the arm rests relaxed on the surface.] ... ... good ... ... very good ... ...

+++ End of Option 2 +++

Distribution, publication, and copying in any form are prohibited and subject to damages.

All Titles in the Series

Volume 1: Smoking Cessation
Volume 2: Anxiety and Restlessness
Volume 3: Burnout
Volume 4: Reducing Overweight
Volume 5: Coping with the Past
Volume 6: Suicidal Thoughts and Attempts
Volume 7: Psycho-Oncology
Volume 8: Obsessions and Tics
Volume 9: Self-Confidence and Decision-Making
Volume 10: Grief Work
Volume 11: Psychosomatics
Volume 12: Chronic Pain
Volume 13: Depressive Thoughts
Volume 14: Panic Attacks
Volume 15: Domestic Violence, Victim Support
Volume 16: Post-Traumatic Stress
Volume 17: Exam Anxiety and Stage Fright
Volume 18: Anti-Violence Training, Offender Support
Volume 19: Addiction Tendencies
Volume 20: Social Phobia and Fear of Contact
Volume 21: Nail Biting
Volume 22: Self-Awareness and Self-Love
Volume 23: Teeth Grinding and Night Clenching
Volume 24: Feelings of Guilt
Volume 25: Fear in Crowds
Volume 26: Fear of Flying, Aviophobia
Volume 27: Fear in Enclosed Spaces, Claustrophobia
Volume 28: Tinnitus, Ear Noises
Volume 29: Fear of Heights
Volume 30: Neurodermatitis

Copying, publishing, and sharing with third parties are only permitted with the written consent of the author. Please observe the notes on copyright and usage.

Volume 31: Finding Inner Balance
Volume 32: Overcoming Loneliness
Volume 33: Fear of Illness, Hypochondria
Volume 34: Anticipatory Anxiety, Fear of Fear
Volume 35: Jealousy in Relationships
Volume 36: Driving Anxiety
Volume 37: New Start after Separation
Volume 38: Fear of Injections
Volume 39: Heart Anxiety Neurosis
Volume 40: Overcoming Resentment and Anger
Volume 41: Resolving Blockages and Positive Thinking
Volume 42: Stress Reduction, Stress Management
Volume 43: Body Relaxation
Volume 44: Deep Relaxation
Volume 45: Fear of the Dark
Volume 46: Falling Asleep and Staying Asleep
Volume 47: Compulsive Buying
Volume 48: Restless Legs Syndrome
Volume 49: Bulimia
Volume 50: Anorexia
Volume 51: Overcoming Nightmares
Volume 52: Imagined Deformity
Volume 53: Overcoming Distrust, Finding Trust
Volume 54: Processing Failures
Volume 55: Humiliation, Emotional Hurt
Volume 56: Distressing Compassion, Vicarious Suffering
Volume 57: Self-Forgiveness
Volume 58: Self-Awareness, Self-Confidence
Volume 59: Saying No
Volume 60: Assertiveness
Volume 61: Setting Boundaries and Self-Assertion
Volume 62: Decision-Making Ability

Volume 63: Success Orientation
Volume 64: Ruminating, Circular Thinking
Volume 65: Accepting Pregnancy
Volume 66: Birth Preparation
Volume 67: Spiritual Opening
Volume 68: Joy of Life and Inner Lightness
Volume 69: Patience and Inner Peace
Volume 70: Fibromyalgia and Rheumatism
Volume 71: Irritable Bowel Syndrome, Crohn's Disease
Volume 72: Fear of Nausea, Emetophobia
Volume 73: Stuttering and Cluttering, Speech Flow Disorders
Volume 74: Concentration and Knowledge Anchoring
Volume 75: Vitality and Spontaneity
Volume 76: Searching for Meaning and Finding Goals
Volume 77: Life Crises, Life Events
Volume 78: Workaholism, Goal Obsession
Volume 79: Helper Syndrome, Helpless Helpers
Volume 80: Medication Abuse
Volume 81: Gambling Addiction
Volume 82: Internet Addiction, Smartphone Addiction
Volume 83: Hoarding Disorder, Compulsive Collecting
Volume 84: Conspiracy Thoughts, Overvalued Ideas
Volume 85: Fear of Operations and Treatments
Volume 86: Fear of Aging
Volume 87: Travel Anxiety
Volume 88: Anxiety When Urinating, Paruresis
Volume 89: Fear of Intimacy and Togetherness
Volume 90: Fear of Blushing
Volume 91: Coming Out in Homosexuality
Volume 92: Charisma Training
Volume 93: Migraines and Chronic Headaches
Volume 94: Overcoming Allergies, Bronchial Asthma

Volume 95: Normalizing Blood Pressure
Volume 96: Compulsive Perfectionism
Volume 97: Sports Hypnosis, Motivation
Volume 98: Sports Hypnosis, Performance Enhancement
Volume 99: Determination and Focus
Volume 100: Encountering the Inner Child
Volume 101: Cravings, Binge Eating
Volume 102: Stimulating Metabolism
Volume 103: Bipolar Mood Swings
Volume 104: Borderline, Identity Crises
Volume 105: Hypomania, Euphoria, Mania
Volume 106: Restlessness, Agitation
Volume 107: Nervous Breakdown
Volume 108: Adjustment Disorders
Volume 109: Self-Alienation, Depersonalization
Volume 110: Ending Self-Pity
Volume 111: Primary Gain of Illness
Volume 112: Secondary Gain of Illness
Volume 113: Bullying, Victim Support
Volume 114: Letting Go of Envy and Jealousy
Volume 115: Fear of Spiders, Arachnophobia
Volume 116: Fear of Dogs or Cats
Volume 117: Fear of Strangers, Xenophobia
Volume 118: Excessive Worries, Generalized Anxiety
Volume 119: Strengthening Sense of Responsibility
Volume 120: Unrequited Love, Heartache
Volume 121: Work-Life Balance
Volume 122: Letting Go of Unattainable Goals
Volume 123: Allowing and Accepting Help
Volume 124: Letting Go of Adult Children
Volume 125: Tourette Syndrome
Volume 126: Life Changes and New Starts

Volume 127: Accepting Life in a Wheelchair
Volume 128: Understanding and Overcoming Homesickness
Volume 129: Understanding and Overcoming Wanderlust
Volume 130: Dizziness, Meniere's Disease
Volume 131: Overcoming Aggression
Volume 132: Cutting and Self-Harm
Volume 133: Hair Pulling, Trichotillomania
Volume 134: Postpartum Depression
Volume 135: For Relatives of Dementia Patients
Volume 136: Self-Harm, Artificial Disorders
Volume 137: Activating Self-Healing Powers
Volume 138: Preventing Depression Relapse
Volume 139: Reactive Psychoses, Follow-Up
Volume 140: Obsessive Thoughts and Impulses
Volume 141: Compulsive Checking
Volume 142: Compulsive Counting, Symmetry Obsession
Volume 143: Compulsive Washing, Cleanliness Obsession
Volume 144: Compulsive Questioning
Volume 145: Dissociative Paralysis
Volume 146: Phantom Pain
Volume 147: Overcoming Complaining
Volume 148: Hay Fever, Pollen Allergy
Volume 149: Sexual Abuse, Victim Support
Volume 150: Standing Strong Against Sexism, #metoo
Volume 151: Binge Eating
Volume 152: Overcoming Thoughts of Revenge
Volume 153: Detachment from the Aggressor, Stockholm Syndrome
Volume 154: Courage to Separate
Volume 155: Chronic Fatigue, Exhaustion
Volume 156: Fear of the Future, Existential Anxiety
Volume 157: Excessive Worry About Children
Volume 158: Fear of Failure

Volume 159: Ending Distrust and Control
Volume 160: Dejection, Dysphoria
Volume 161: Boreout, Chronic Boredom
Volume 162: Bipolar Disorders, Relapse Prevention
Volume 163: Mania, Relapse Prevention
Volume 164: Nihilism, Feelings of Worthlessness
Volume 165: Thumb Sucking
Volume 166: Being Brave
Volume 167: Being Proud
Volume 168: Overcoming Shyness
Volume 169: Being Able to Delegate Responsibility
Volume 170: Being Able to Show Emotions
Volume 171: Letting Go of Guilt, Victim Support
Volume 172: Processing Guilt, Offender Support
Volume 173: Mood Swings, Cyclothymia
Volume 174: Lack of Drive, Vital Sadness
Volume 175: Hearing Voices with Reality Reference
Volume 176: Confident Communication
Volume 177: Standing Up for Oneself
Volume 178: Taking New Paths
Volume 179: Confident Job Application
Volume 180: No Longer Being Taken Advantage Of
Volume 181: End of Submissiveness
Volume 182: Depressive Numbness
Volume 183: Mood Drops, Affective Incontinence
Volume 184: Mood Instability
Volume 185: Somatoform Disorders
Volume 186: Stomach Ulcer, Psychosomatic
Volume 187: Accepting Amputation
Volume 188: Overcoming and Letting Go of Hatred
Volume 189: Ending Accusations
Volume 190: Allowing Tears, Being Able to Cry

Volume 191: Finding and Sorting Repressed Feelings
Volume 192: Somatoform Pain
Volume 193: Living Autonomously
Volume 194: Anhedonia, Joylessness
Volume 195: Persistent Sadness
Volume 196: Obesity, Food Addiction
Volume 197: Parents of Abused Children
Volume 198: Letting Go and Letting Be
Volume 199: Childhood Sexual Abuse
Volume 200: Fear of Loss

www.ingramcontent.com/pod-product-compliance
Lightning Source LLC
Chambersburg PA
CBHW030452220526
45464CB00006B/2506